HENRY'S ZIPPER

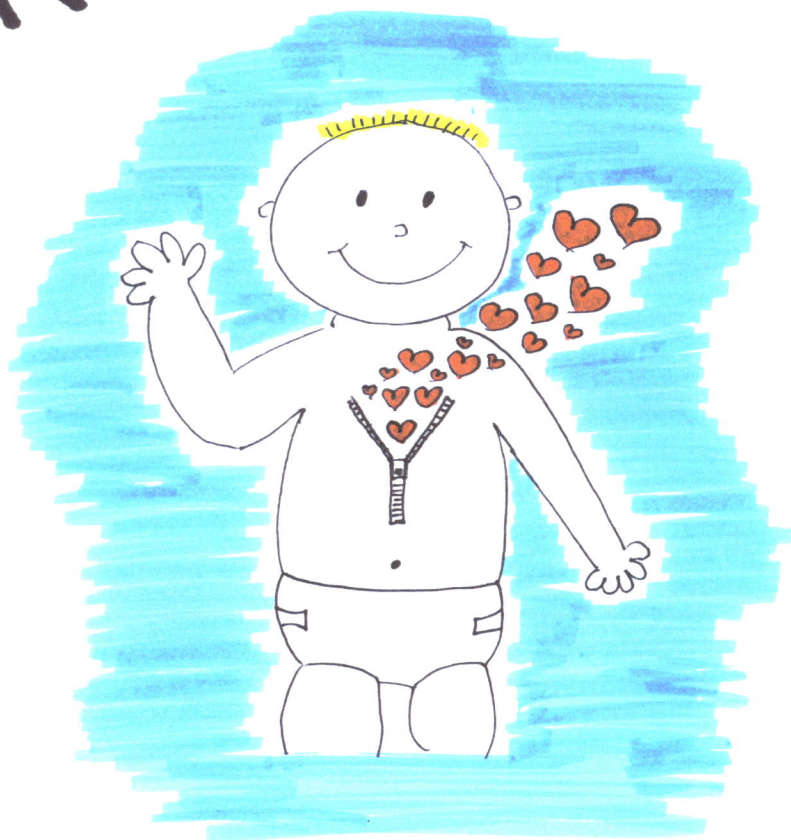

Written and Illustrated by Maureen Horvath

Henry's Zipper

978-1-7336538-0-0 (paperback)
978-1-7336538-1-7 (hardcover)

Published by Heart of Nature Press, Truckee, California

Publisher@HeartofNaturePress.com

The author of this book does not dispense medical advice or prescribe the use of any technique as a form of treatment for physical or medical problems without the advice of a physician, either directly or indirectly. The intent of the author is only to offer information of a general nature to help you in your quest for emotional and spiritual well-being.

This book is for Henry's big sister Evelyn
who always loves with her whole heart.

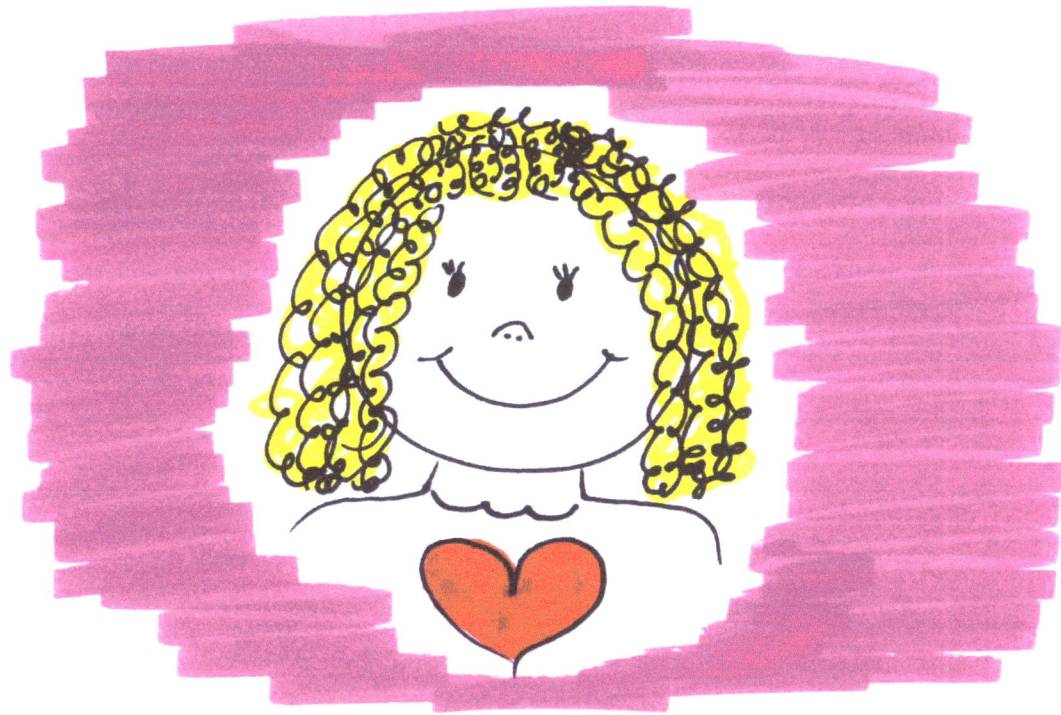

This is Henry.

Henry is a baby.

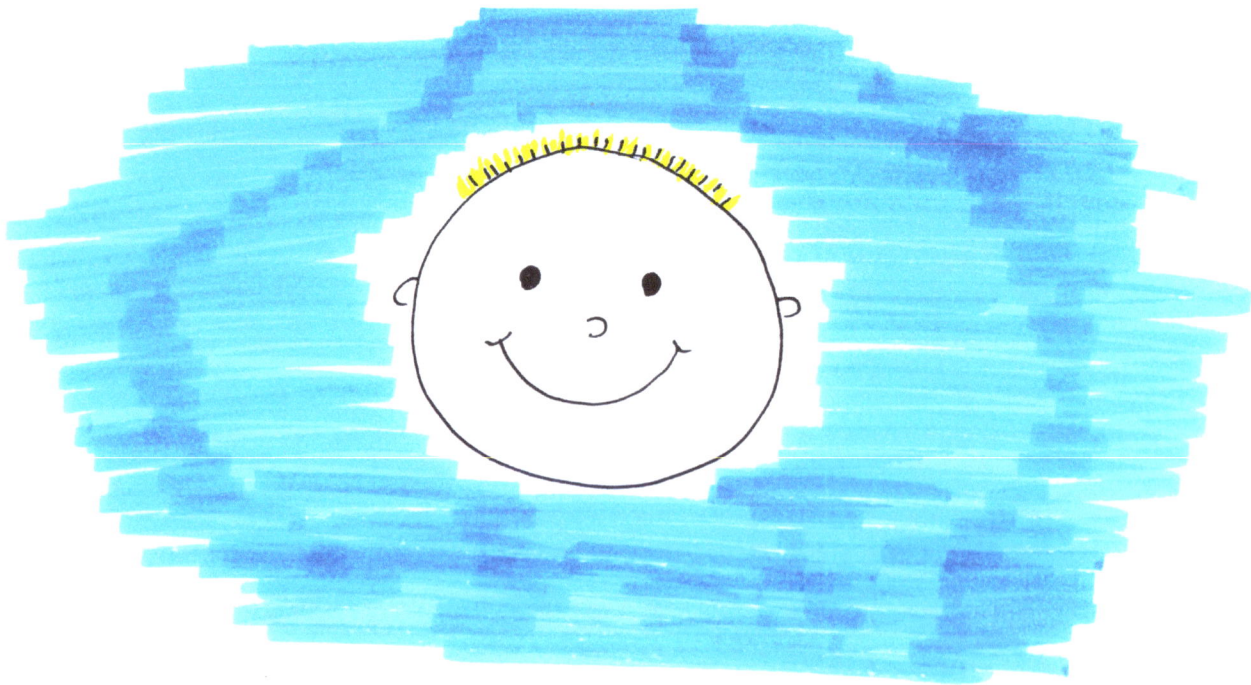

When Henry was only 3 weeks old, the doctor found a hole in his heart.

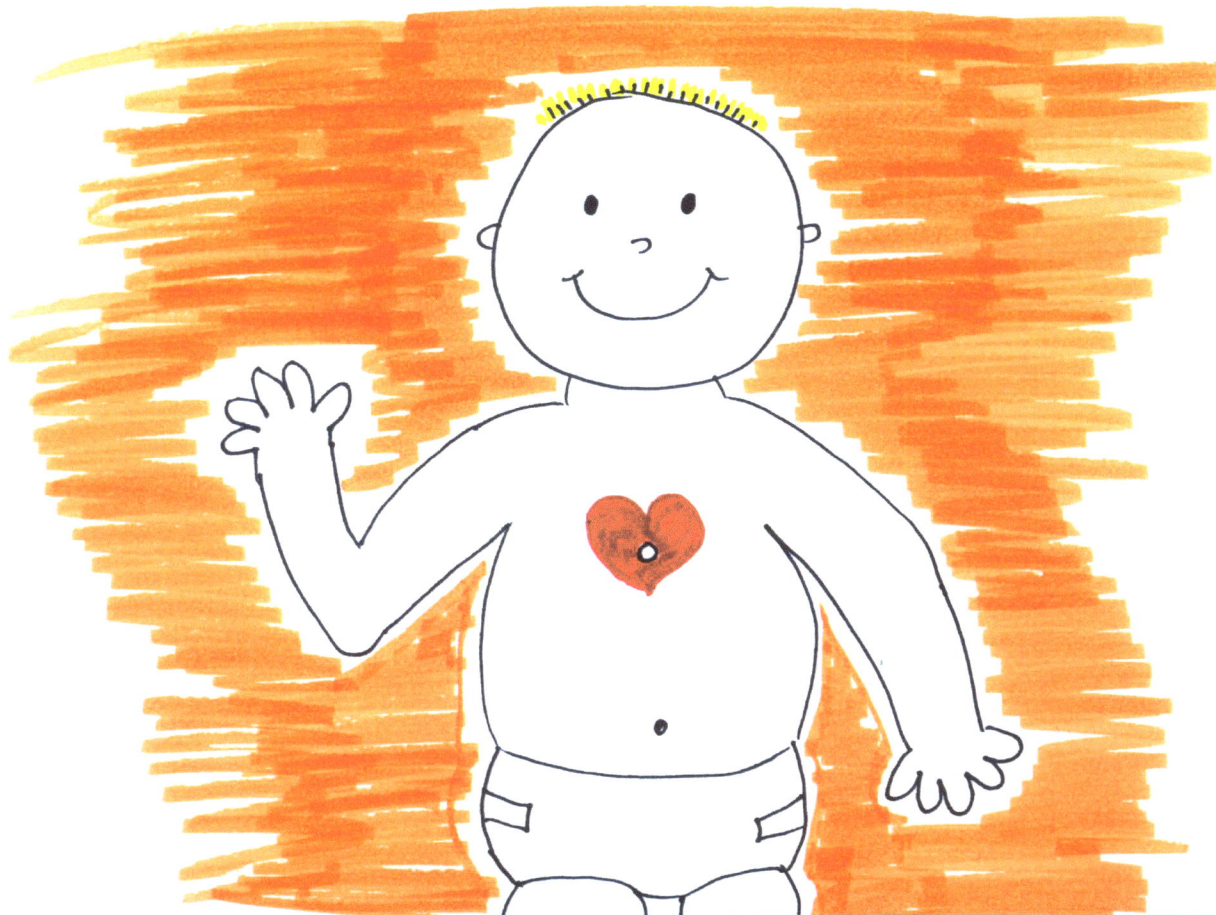

Henry's heart didn't work very well with a hole in it.

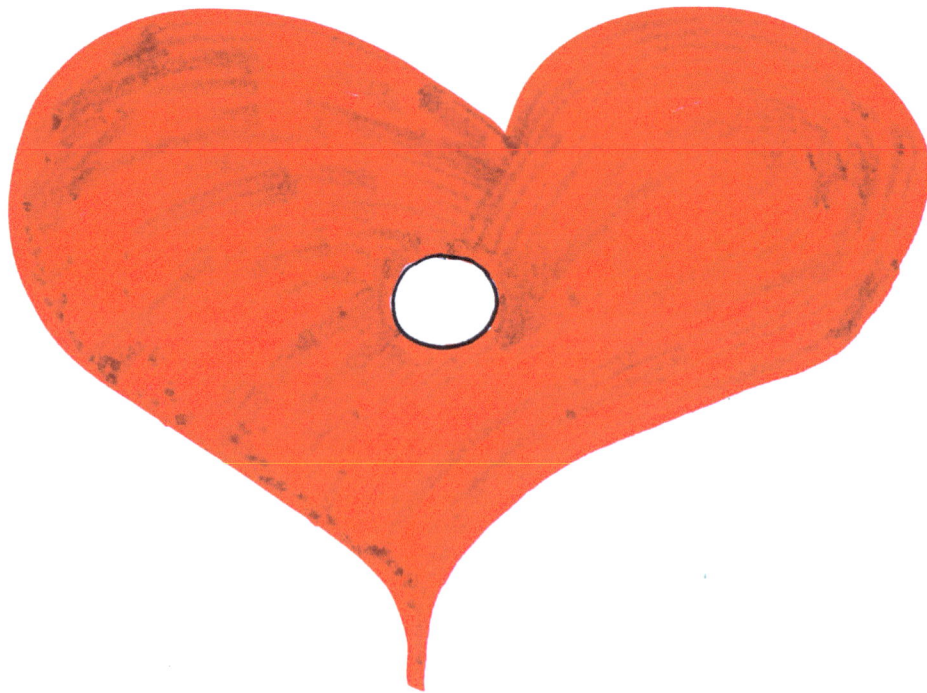

Henry was happy, but the doctors were not happy knowing that there was a hole in his heart.

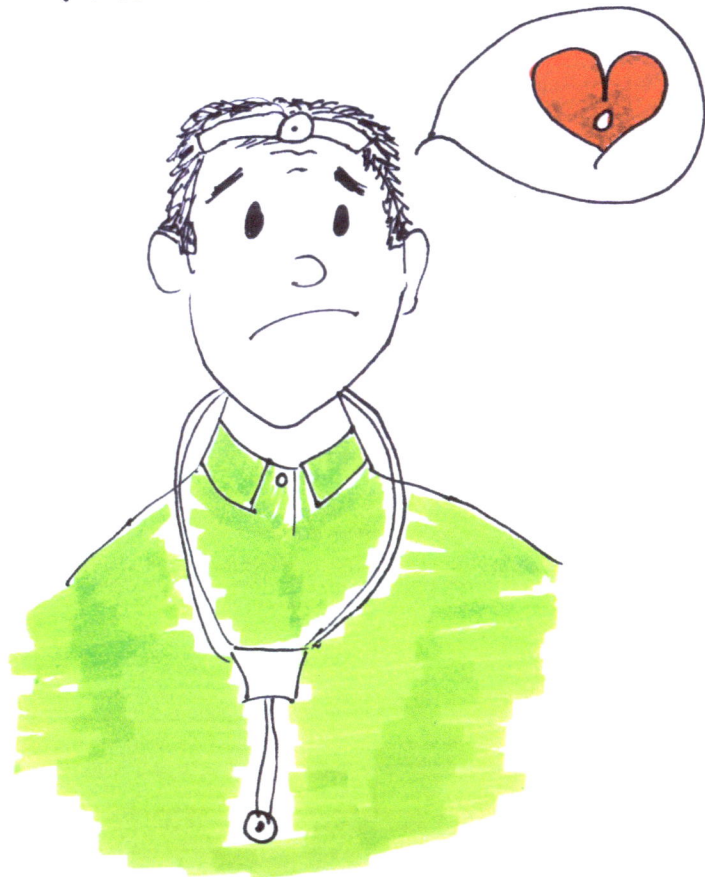

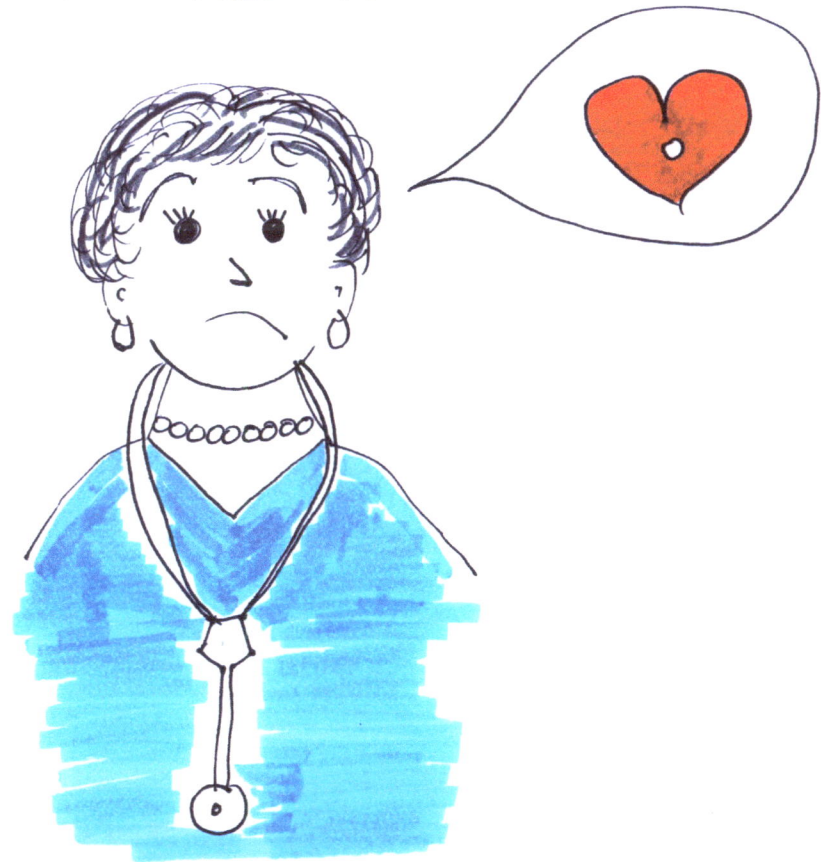

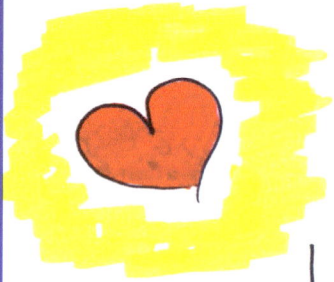

Henry didn't look sick, he even smiled for his mommy, daddy and his big sister Evelyn. Henry liked to grin at their dog Ollie too. There was a lot of love in their family.

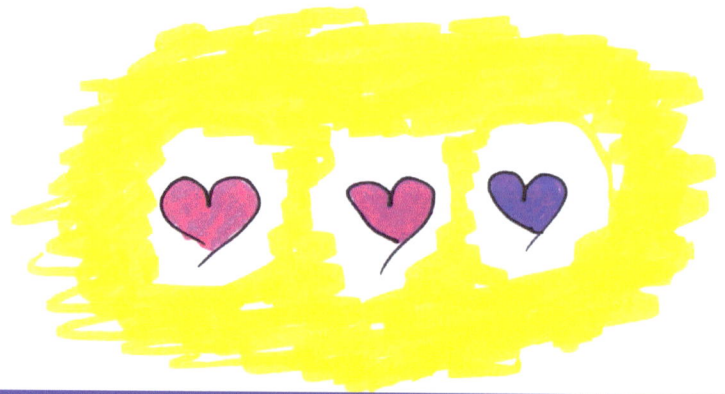

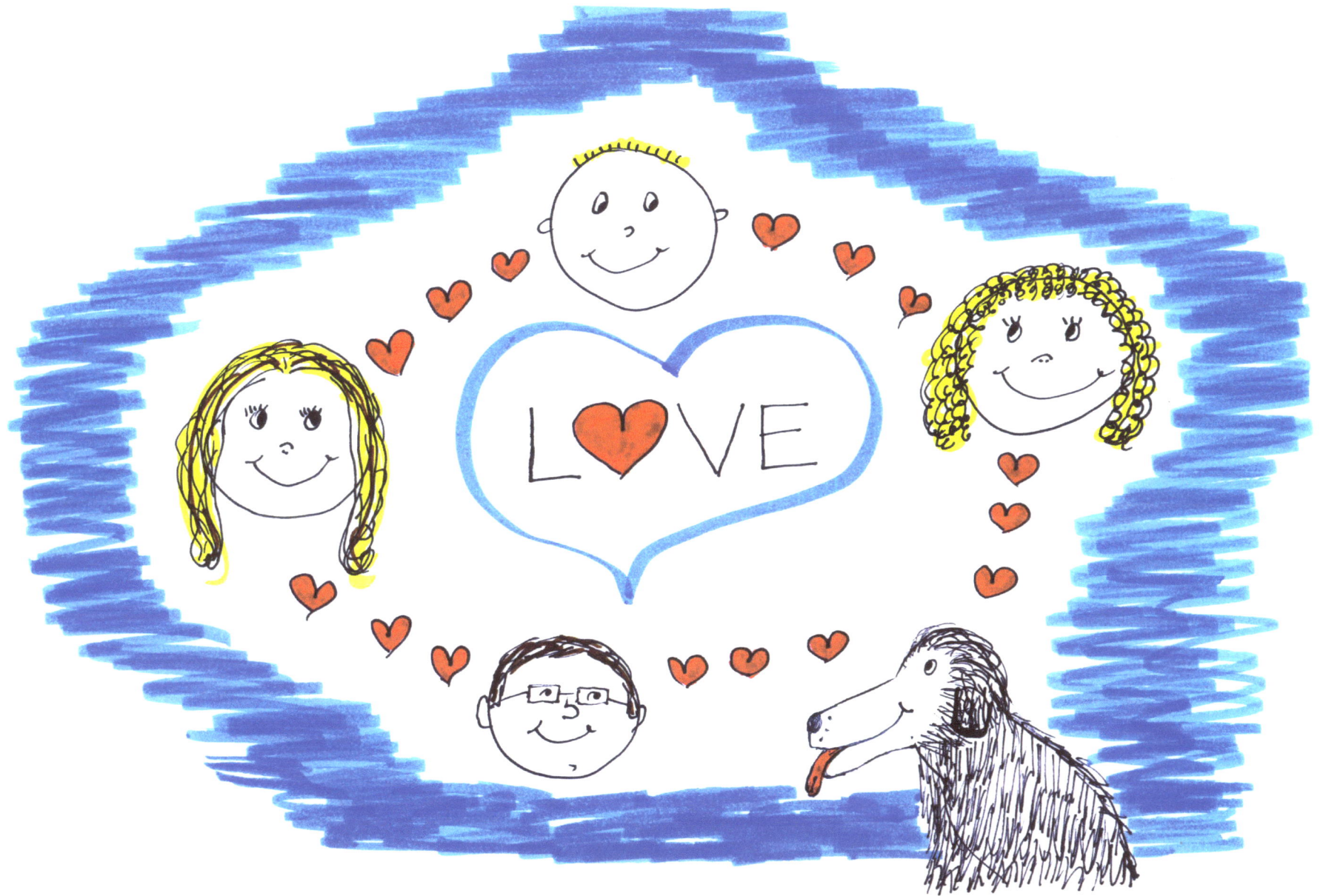

So, Henry had to go to the hospital
and the doctors had to fix his heart.

Mommy, daddy and Evelyn were worried...

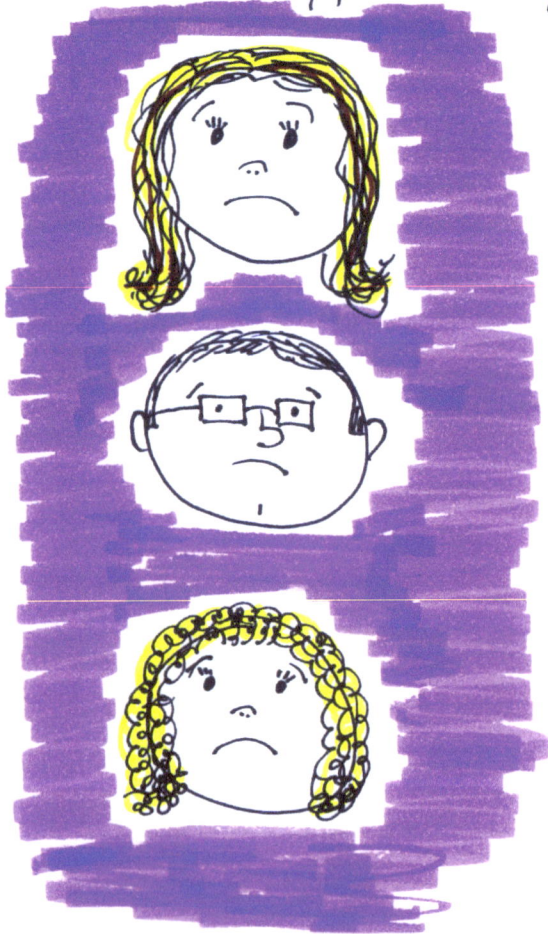

... but Henry wasn't worried

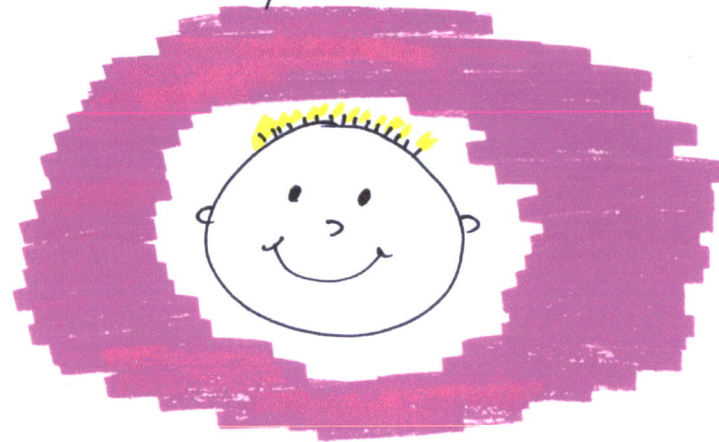

because Henry was a baby and
babies don't know about hospitals.

Hospitals can be scary because some people wear masks and look sick or worried.

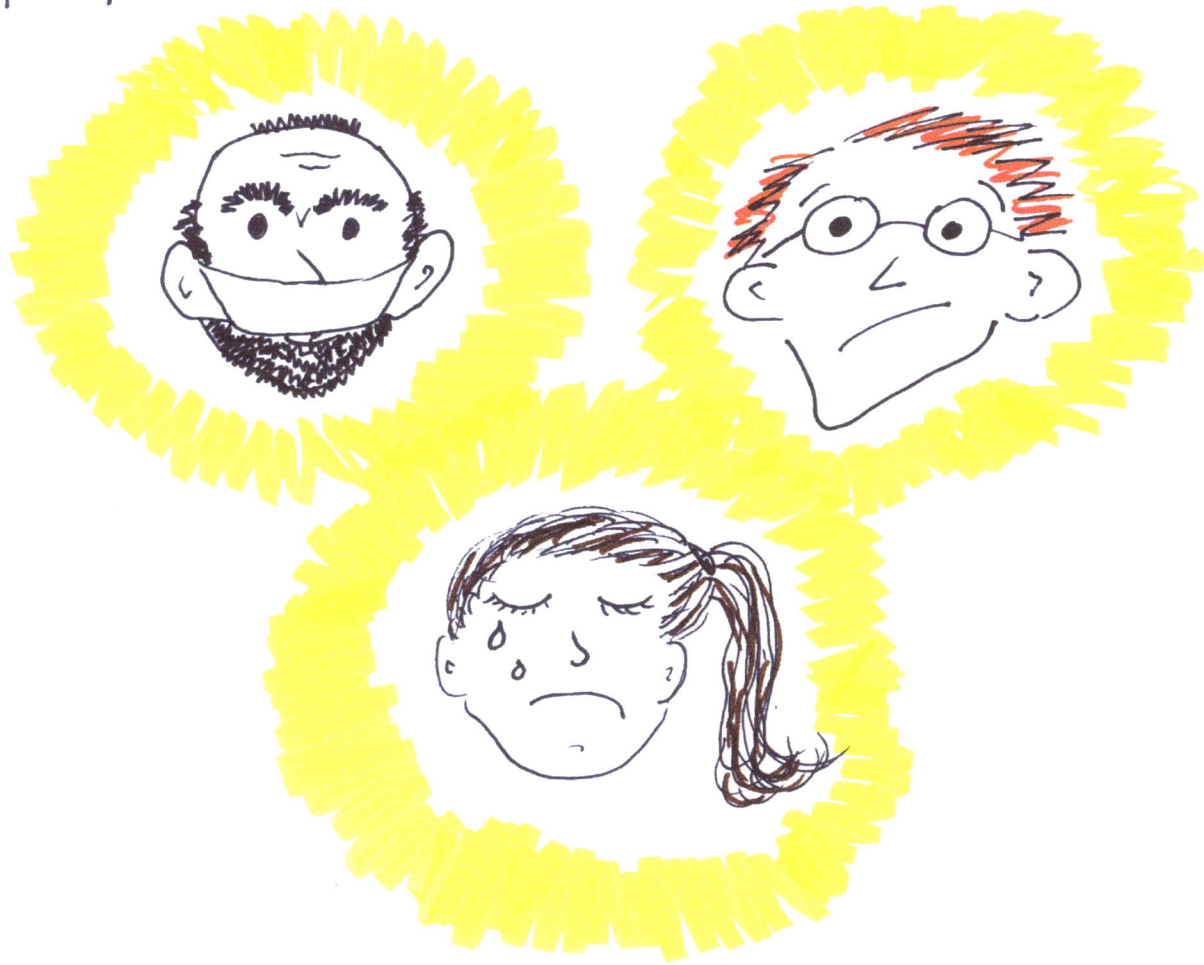

Henry's grandparents, cousins, friends and even friends of friends were very worried for Henry.

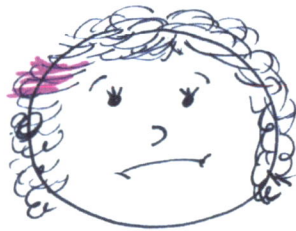

Grandma

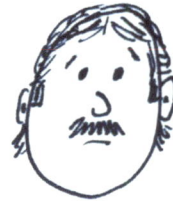

Bampa

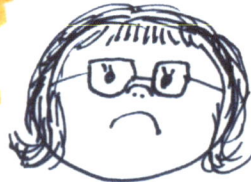

Momo

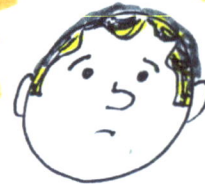

GrandBob

Henry's worried cousins

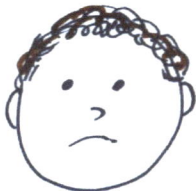
Jakob

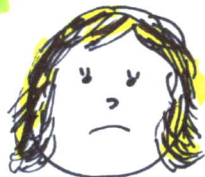
Izabelle

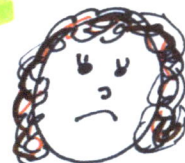
Amelia

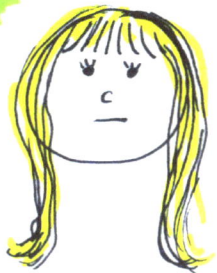
Harper

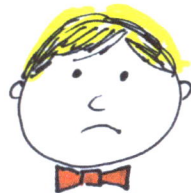
Hudson

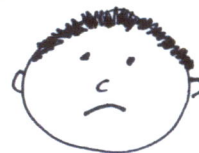
Kingston

People from all over the country sent Henry healing thoughts and prayers. People who didn't even know Henry were hoping his heart would be fixed.

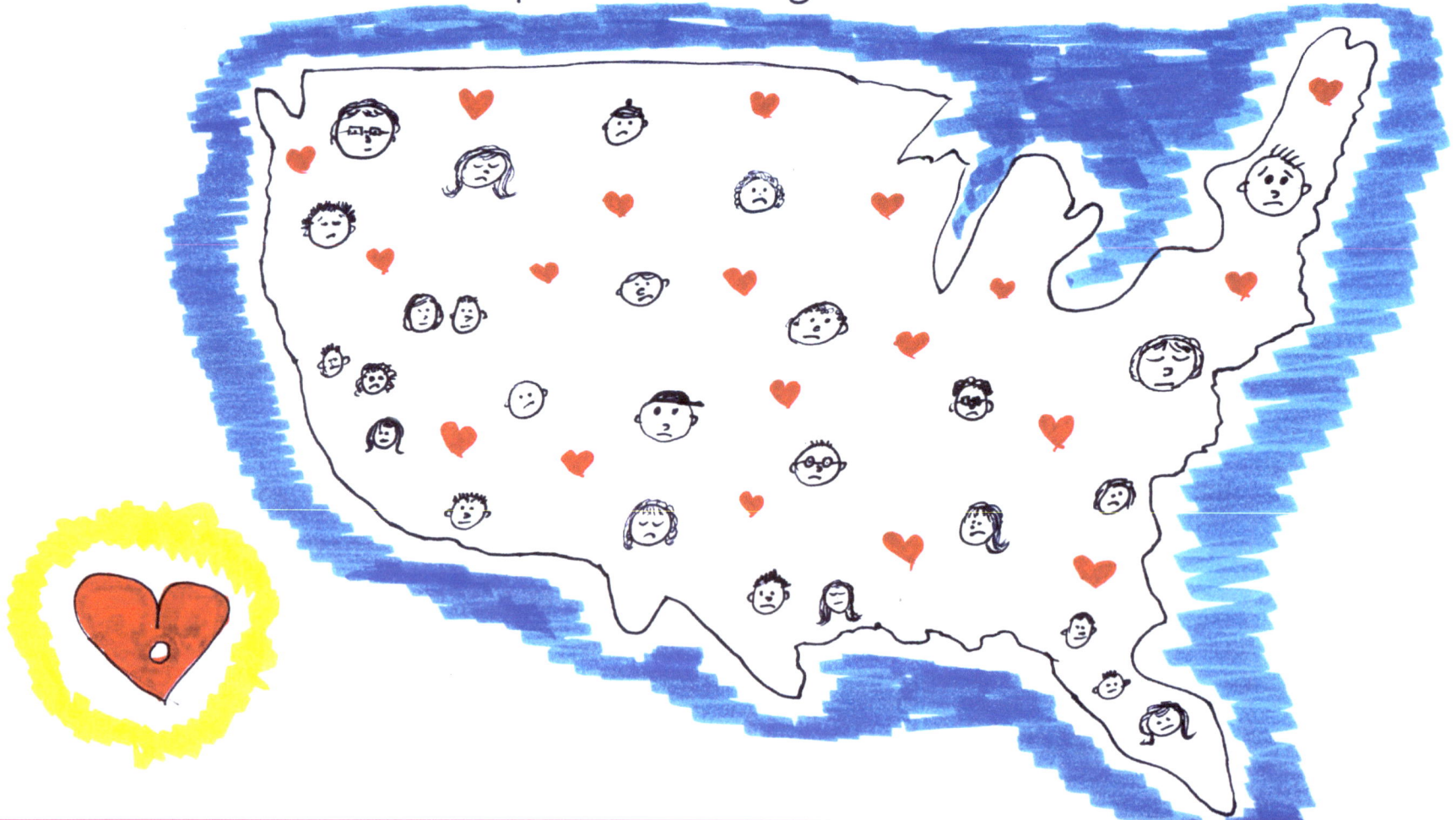

The doctors and nurses at the hospital told
Henry's mommy, daddy and Evelyn that they
would do their best to fix Henry's heart.
To fix the hole, they would have to open his chest.

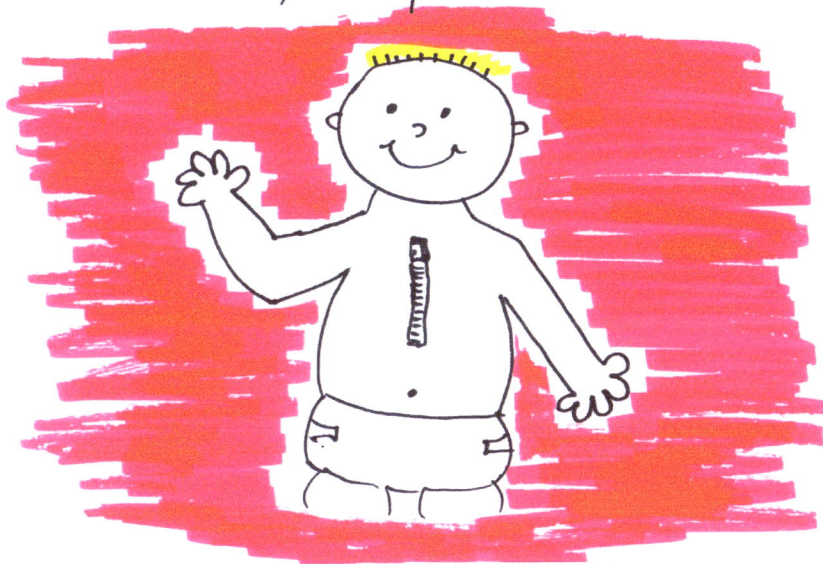

Henry would have a scar on his chest that kind of
looked like a zipper... but it didn't zip or unzip.

At first Henry's zipper looked kind of scary.
Evelyn was afraid it would unzip and his
love would spill out of his chest.

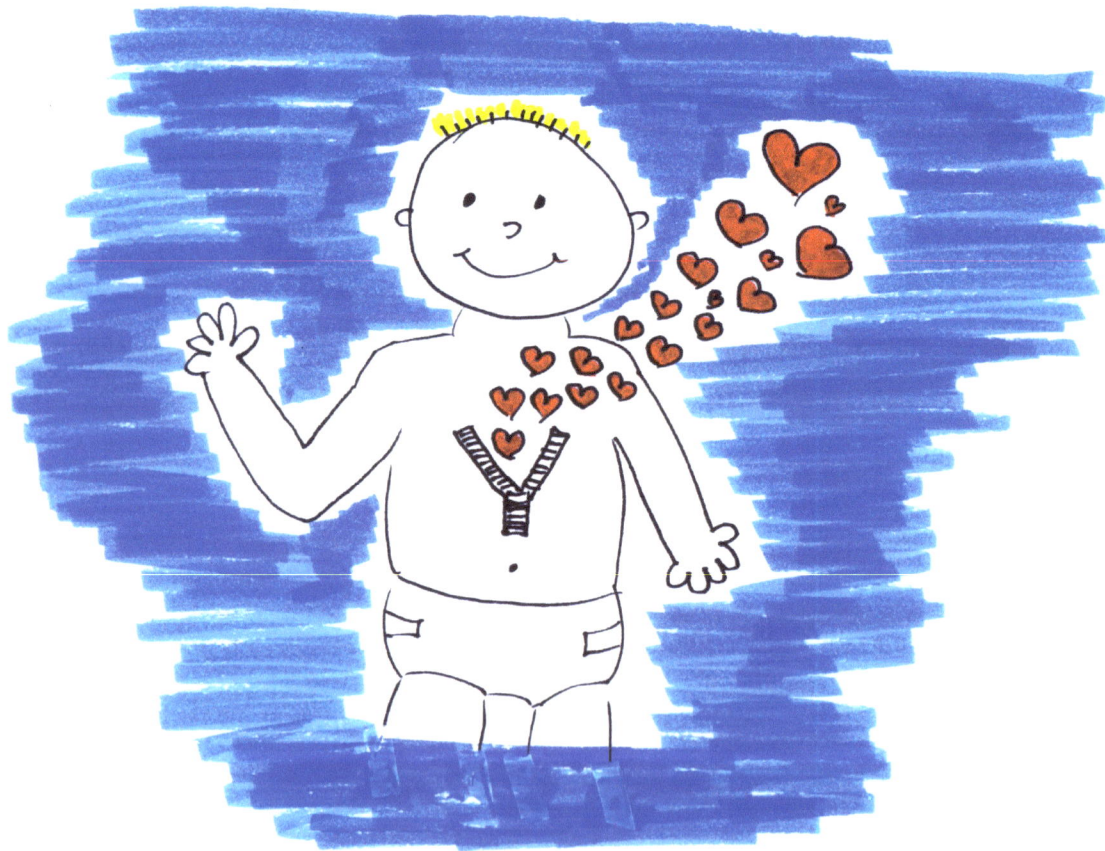

Henry was in the hospital for only one week. The doctors and nurses took care of Henry so well that he came home smiling. Evelyn wasn't afraid of Henry's zipper scar anymore because her family was home again and they were happy together.

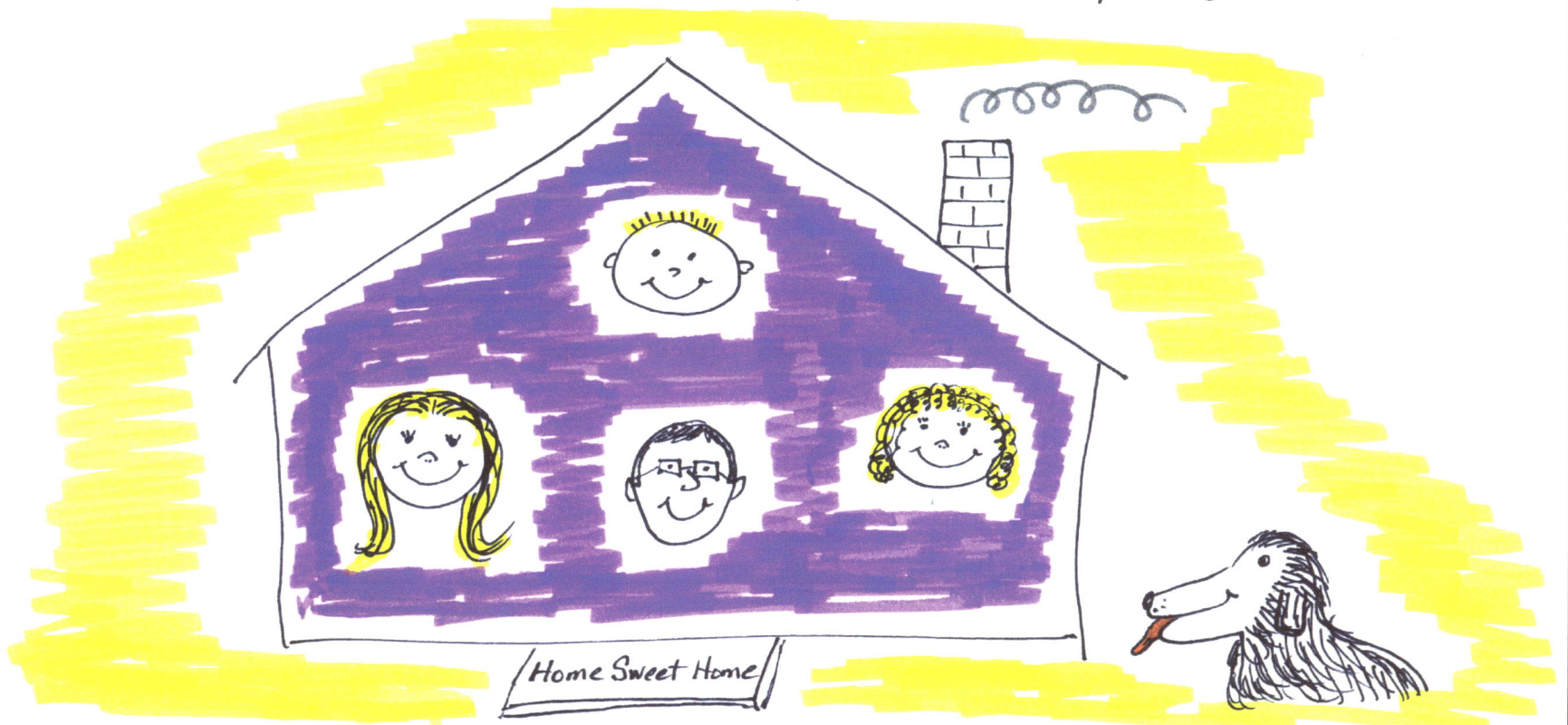

Home Sweet Home

The doctors fixed Henry's hole in his heart and Henry let his love spill out to share with the world. Henry can now love with his _whole_ heart!

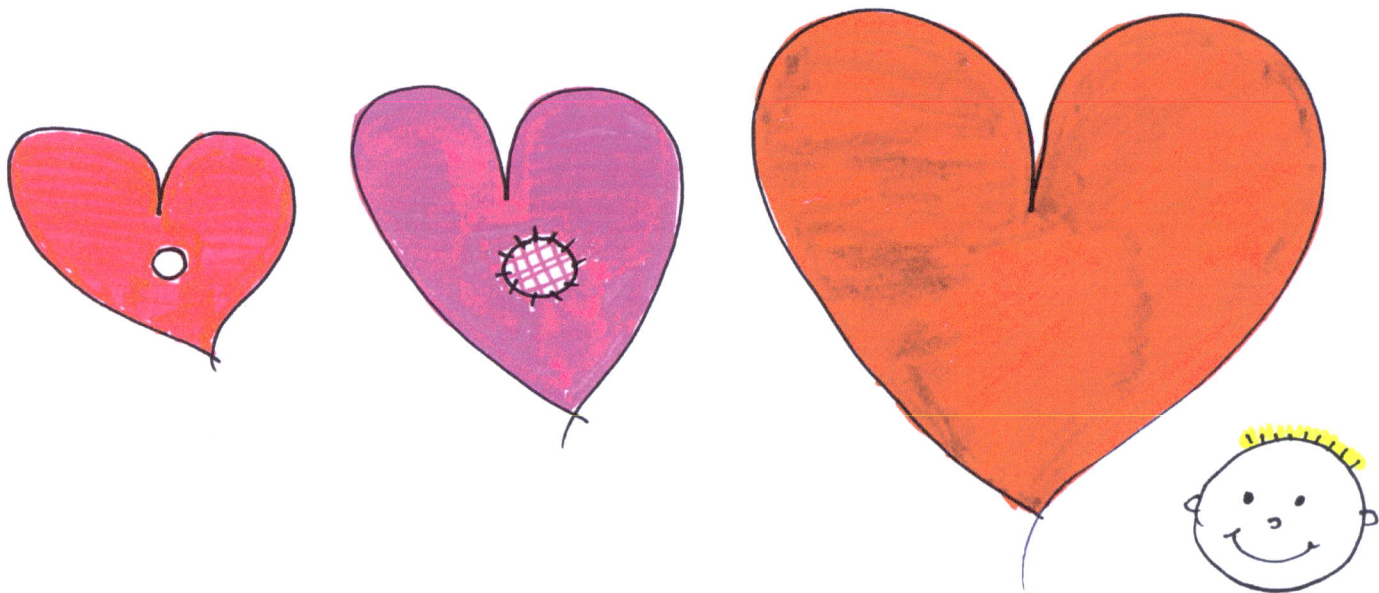

The End

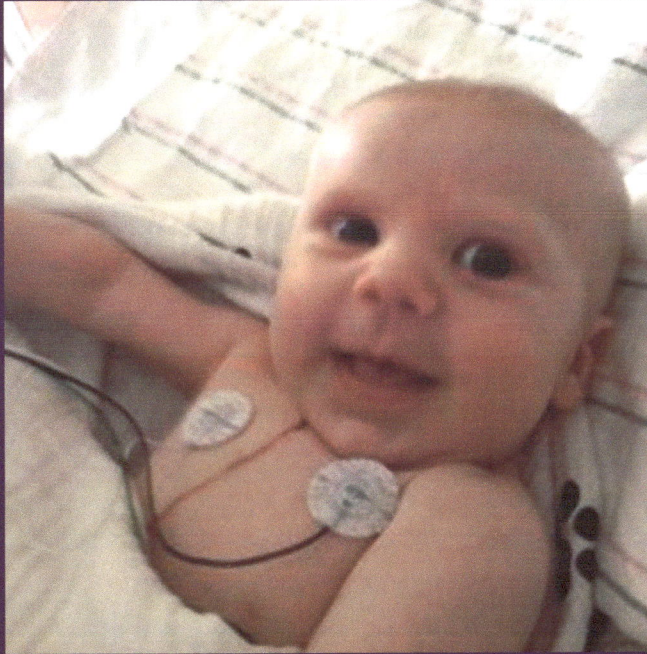

Hi! I'm the "real" Henry! Can you see my zipper? I'm happy that my heart is fixed and I'm going to grow up to be a big boy who can do ANYTHING!

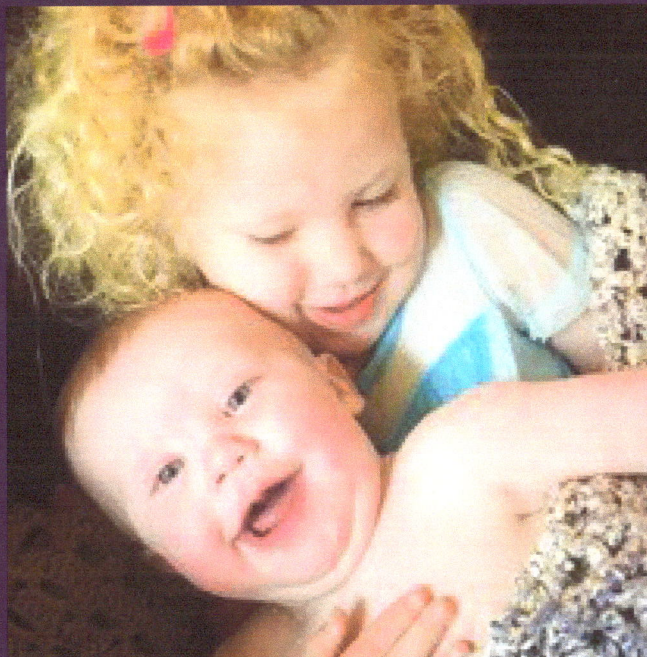

Hi! I'm the real "Evelyn"! I'm so happy that doctors fixed my baby brother Henry. I can't wait until he can walk and talk and play with me. When Henry is older I will tell him about his zipper. I love my family and my brother so much!

Henry's Zipper

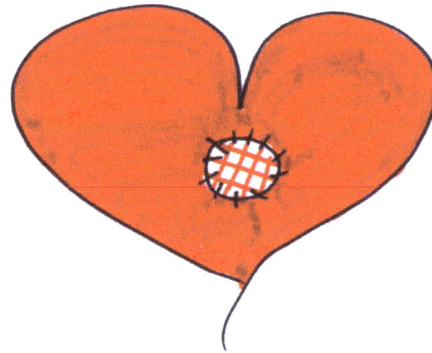

With heartfelt thanks to Dr. Christopher Arth of Truckee, California who first diagnosed Henry and to Dr. Katrinka Kip of Reno, Nevada who referred us to Stanford Medical Center.

And to Dr. Frank Hanley and the remarkable doctors, nurses and staff at Lucile Packard Children's Hospital, we are in awe of your skill, dedication and the caring support of our entire family.